Discover the Beauty of

Self-Love

...Unleashing Your Brilliance, Embracing Your Worth!...

Discover The Beauty of

Self-Love

...Experiencing the Beauty of Self Love...

For more information contact:

Phone; +254 72283 5564/+254-7246 57794

Email :kiruuz@gmail.com

ISBN:
9798879590609

Table of Contents

References:

Introduction.

Welcome to a transformative journey of self-love—a journey that transcends the boundaries of time, culture, and circumstance to touch the depths of our souls and reveal the path to deep personal fulfillment. In a world often filled with demands, expectations, and comparisons, the concept of self-love stands as a beacon of hope—a reminder that there is a deeper connection that can be made amidst life's challenges and what we have with each other. This book is a heartfelt invitation—a gentle nudge to begin a journey of self-discovery and compassion. It is a testament to the belief that within each of us, there is an infinite amount of love, acceptance, and resilience waiting to be tapped. In these pages you will find a mosaic of meditative insights and practical tools designed to guide you on the path to greater self-understanding and acceptance from letting go of self-doubt to fully accepting your emotions, each chapter is designed to support you as you navigate your inner land But this book is more than just the words on the page—it's an invitation to dive deeper, to explore the recesses of the heart with passion and compassion. It's an opportunity to rewrite your story of competence and personality to challenge the narrative that no longer serves you. Traveling through these pages reminds you of the inner beauty and uniqueness that lies within you. As much as you are, take comfort in the understanding that your worthiness is not based on external credentials or perfection Above all, may you realize that the road to self-love is not perfection but where you are—the daily practice of showing up for yourself with kindness, grace, and truth. Embrace the journey with an open heart and curiosity, knowing that every step you take brings you closer to the radiant essence of your being So, dear reader, I invite you to embark on this journey with courage and confidence. Let these words be a guiding light as you navigate your inner wonderland. Leave this journey with love, acceptance, and deep respect for the beautiful soul you are.

Chapter One

Specifying self-love.

In our deeper exploration of our love, we have delved into the intricate details of this transformative journey, searching not only for vague ideas but for deep and defined personal meaning specific to what self-love means. At the heart of this journey is the realization that self-love is a dynamic and transformative force, unique to each individual. This is not a one-size-fits-all perspective but rather a deeply personal commitment to understanding, embracing, and equally accepting all aspects—faults, quirks, strengths, and weaknesses. Within the fabric of self-love lies the need for self-awareness—and unexamined look into our deepest thoughts, feelings, and beliefs. This self-knowledge becomes a compass that guides us toward truth, motivating us to set aside life's expectations and embrace our true selves. An important aspect is evident in their self-acceptance. Not only does it acknowledge our existence, it also fully embraces the essence of who we are. This includes making peace with our imperfections, letting go of the chains of self-esteem, and celebrating the unique fabric that defines our individuality

Embedded in this insight is the concept of healthy boundaries—the cornerstone of self-love. It's about recognizing our flaws, learning to say no when necessary, and putting our best interests first without guilt or apology.

By defining these boundaries, we create a space where self-love can flourish without ceasing. Their pity flows through the story like a gentle stream. To extend kindness to ourselves in times of struggle, understanding that mistakes are part of the human experience, means treating ourselves with the same warmth and understanding we give to a dear friend. It is a constant process that fosters compassionate dialogue among them and fosters an atmosphere of unconditional helpfulness among us.

The insight reveals the transformative power of self-care—not just as a routine but as a profound act of self-love. This includes listening to our physical and emotional needs, nourishing ourselves with activities that bring happiness, and recognizing that putting our well-being first is not selfish but fundamental to celebrating the temple that lies ahead.

Embedded in this journey is that self-love extends beyond individual identity, and inserts itself into the wider fabric of relationships.

This includes finding the right relationships and setting standards for how much we allow ourselves to heal, by surrounding ourselves with those who nurture and appreciate who we are. As we navigate the complexity of self-love, let us discover the concept of forgiveness—a bandage for the wounds of the past. Not just forgiving others but, perhaps more profoundly, forgiving yourself. It's a journey to let go of the burden that is the weight of our spirit and to open the way for growth and renewal.

Essentially, self-love goes beyond mere definition; This complex mosaic, personal journey that includes self-discovery, acceptance, healthy boundaries, self-compassion, self-care, meaningful relationships, and forgiveness is an ongoing quest, a nuanced one that invites us to continually redefine and refine our understanding of this depth and transformative potential.

Chapter Two

Checking Out Self-Awareness

In the complete exploration of self-attention, we delve into the tricky layers of consciousness, inviting a deep and nuanced expertise of this foundational pillar in the adventure of self-discovery and private growth.

At its essence, self-cognizance is the introspective gaze into the inner workings of our thoughts, emotions, and ideals. It is going beyond the floor, urging us to emerge as attuned to the subtle nuances of our reactions, desires, and motivations. This journey of self-attention unfolds as an ongoing talk with the self—a profound exploration into the middle of our being. Within this expansive exploration lies the popularity that self-cognizance is not a static state but a dynamic procedure. It involves a non-stop dedication to watching, thinking, and knowing the ever-transferring panorama of our internal global. It's an exercise of turning into intimacy with the intricacies of our minds and hearts, unraveling the layers that make contributions to the tapestry of our particular selves.

A pivotal facet of self-recognition is the potential to study without judgment. It involves cultivating a non-crucial focus, permitting the mind and emotions to surface without condemnation. This mild remark creates a safe area for self-exploration, fostering a compassionate know-how of the complexities that shape our thoughts and behaviors.

As we navigate the landscape of self-cognizance, we come across the reflection of the mirrored image—a device that aids in knowledge of the styles, inclinations, and reactions that outline our identity. This replicate activates us to inquire into the origins of our beliefs, hard assumptions, and biases that can be ingrained over time.

Simultaneously, self-attention invites the exploration of our values and dreams. It beckons us to align our actions with our authentic selves, fostering an experience of congruence between our inner landscape and outside expressions. In this alignment, we find out a profound authenticity—a harmony that resonates with the core of our being. A primary theme woven into the cloth of self-awareness is the interconnectedness between mind and frame.

The exploration extends beyond the cognitive realm, recognizing the understanding housed in bodily sensations and emotions. The integration of thoughts-body awareness turns into a gateway to holistic well-being, unraveling the symbiotic relationship between our mental and physical states. In this intricate journey, self-recognition unveils its role as a catalyst for boom and transformation. It empowers us to apprehend regions for improvement, inspiring a dedication to continual mastering and evolution.

Through self-attention, we emerge as architects of our improvement, sculpting a route that aligns with our aspirations and values. As we finish this deep dive into self-recognition, it is evident that this exploration is not a destination but a lifelong odyssey—an ongoing conversation with the self that unfolds with each passing moment. It's an intimate dance with our essence, an embodiment of the complexities that make us beautifully human.

In the dynamics of self-awareness, the threads of introspection, commentary, non-judgmental recognition, mirrored image, alignment, mind-body connection, and increase intricately weave together, crafting a story of profound self-discovery and empowerment. In the profound journey of self-discovery, the exploration of recognizing strengths and weaknesses emerges as a cornerstone, inviting individuals to embark on a deep and introspective inquiry into the facets that shape their identities.

At its essence, spotting strengths includes a deliberate and honest exam of the features, skills, and capabilities that define a person's strong point. It is a celebration of innate gifts—an aware acknowledgment of the abilities and attributes that contribute to individuality.

This method goes beyond an insignificant superficial stock, delving into the reservoir of ability, and inspiring people to embrace and leverage their strengths in numerous life domain names. Simultaneously, the exploration extends to the realm of weaknesses—a terrain frequently approached with hesitation. Instead of viewing weaknesses as flaws, this adventure encourages people to technique them with interest and reputation.

Weaknesses are not indicators of inadequacy however regions of boom and improvement, provide possibilities for getting to know, refinement, and resilience. It's an invitation to recognize and navigate the aspects that gift challenges, fostering a compassionate understanding of obstacles.

Central to this exploration is the cultivation of self-compassion—a gentle acknowledgment that human beings are complicated tapestries of strengths and weaknesses. Through self-compassion, individuals navigate the terrain with kindness, recognizing that imperfections contribute to the richness of human enjoyment.

The system entails a deep dive into narratives—the tales individuals inform themselves about who they are and what they can reap. These narratives form self-belief, influencing the lens through which strengths and weaknesses are viewed. Through introspection, people unveil narratives that empower and uplift even as figuring out the ones that can restrict potential. This focus turns into a device for reshaping self-communicating and fostering an attitude that amplifies strengths and embraces vulnerabilities.

In this exploration, the interconnectedness among strengths and weaknesses will become obtrusive. Strengths remove darkness from the route toward self-success, while weaknesses, approached with humility and a boom attitude, become stepping stones for non-public development.

The journey encourages a dynamic dance among those factors, fostering balanced self-cognizance that transcends societal expectations. As individuals navigate the terrain of spotting strengths and weaknesses, the adventure isn't always certainly one of assessment or judgment but an intimate communication with the self. It's an ongoing technique of self-reflection, taking into consideration evolution and redefinition of what it way to be robust, capable, and authentically human.

In this discourse, individuals unveil the kaleidoscope of being, embracing both the brilliance of strengths and the mosaic of weaknesses with grace, resilience, and an unwavering dedication to chronic boom. In the tremendous panorama of self-discovery and personal growth, authenticity emerges as a guiding principle—a beacon that illuminates the direction toward deeper understanding and acceptance of oneself.

At its middle, authenticity beckons people to embody and encompass their true essence—their ideals, values, passions, and quirks—without pretense or conformity to external expectations. It is an invitation to strip away the mask we put on, revealing the raw, unfiltered fact of who we are underneath the layers of societal conditioning and cultural norms. Authenticity starts to evolve with a profound adventure inward—an exploration of the internal landscape where our private truths are living.

It calls for radical self-honesty, a willingness to confront the parts of ourselves we may also opt to preserve hidden or suppressed. Through introspection and reflection, we discover the essence of our being—the core truths that outline our identity and form our lived revel. This journey of self-discovery isn't always usually smooth. It requires courage to embrace vulnerability—to expose our true selves to the arena, knowing that we can be met with judgment, rejection, or false impressions.

Yet, it is through this vulnerability that true connection and intimacy are forged, as others are invited to witness and have fun with the authenticity of our being. Authenticity also entails living in alignment with our values and ideals, even in the face of adversity or societal strain to conform. It requires courage to face firm in our convictions, to talk about our reality, and to honor the dictates of our judgment of right and wrong, even if it approaches swimming in opposition to the present-day popular opinion. Moreover, authenticity invites an experience of wholeness and integration—a harmonious alignment of our inner and outer selves.

It entails honoring the myriad dimensions of our identification—the mild and the shadow, the strengths, and the vulnerabilities—and embracing them as imperative aspects of our humanity. In cultivating authenticity, we allow ourselves to live authentically—to express ourselves freely, to pursue our passions wholeheartedly, and to forge meaningful connections primarily based on true mutual information and recognition. It is through this authenticity that we find authentic success and belonging, as we honor the precise items and contributions that every folk brings to the tapestry of human enjoyment. In essence, authenticity isn't always a vacation spot to be reached however a lifelong adventure—an ongoing manner of self-discovery and self-expression.

It is a commitment to residing with integrity, congruence, and courage—to being real to ourselves and to the essence of who we are, regardless of where the adventure may lead.

Chapter Three

Nurturing Self-Compassion

In the ride in the direction of self-love assisting self-compassion involves an essential turning point. Within the midst of our internal discussion exists the danger of growing generosity plus knowledge within the direction of ourselves. Right here, we find out the vast significance of self-compassion and also its transformative energy.

Self-compassion, at its middle, has to do with prolonging equal warmth, remedy along help to ourselves that we comfortably supply to others. It starts with spotting our very personal mankind, with all its blemishes in addition to susceptibilities. In mins of struggle, failure, or soreness self-compassion permits us to keep ourselves with infection together with approval. Sometimes the globe around us would possibly resemble assumptions of excellence urging us to perform even extra alongside be plenty higher.

Nevertheless, self-compassion welcomes us to welcome our blemishes as a thing of our common mankind. It advises us that we deserve love as well as coming from, no matter our issues, however because of them. Cultivating self-compassion requires a moderate lifestyle of mind, based totally on mindfulness. By adjusting properly to the present minute with inquisitiveness and also visibility we will look at our thoughts coupled with feelings without judgment. Via mindfulness strategies we find out to welcome the complete variety of our inner reviews, promoting a considerate reputation of ourselves.

In the method of self-compassion, self-kindness arises as a supporting light. It urges us to visit ourselves with the same meekness in addition to the motivation we offer to bosom friends. Via acts of self-kindness whether or not with affirmations, self-care workouts or merely prolonging a relaxing contact we guide the seeds of compassion within.

Vital to self-compassion is the acknowledgment of our usual humankind. In mins of misery, it's far too clean to sense separation in our battles.
Nonetheless, acknowledging that suffering is a critical element of the human problem promotes a sense of link coupled with belonging. We understand that we are not the most effective ones in our studies; we're certain that each other is different through our commonplace pleasures and also grief fulfillment coupled with challenges.

Supporting self-compassion is not regarding removing all traces of self-complaint or adverse self-communicate. Instead, it consists of growing a thoughtful action to our inner battles. When confronted with self-doubt or objection we can carefully advocate ourselves of our fundamental well worth in addition to worth, accepting ourselves with authentic approval.

Incorporating self-compassion right into our ordinary lives requires cause plus technique. It entails creating an awareness initiative to be cognizant of self-kindness in our ideas and activities. As we browse the intricacies of existence self-compassion becomes our unfaltering pal, providing relief as well as help inside the middle of the ebb plus move of presence.

In supporting self-compassion, we begin a profound ride of self-discovery plus recuperation. We find out to befriend ourselves with genuine compassion as well as information growing a deep feeling of love and approval from inside. With the mild welcome of self-compassion, we awaken to the essential allure coupled with the power of our actual selves. Exercising Self-Kindness: Within the greater comprehensive phase of nurturing Self-Compassion, & quote; exists the crucial quarter of practicing Self-Kindness.

Below we dig right into the art of treating ourselves with warm temperature, and expertise alongside meekness-- a keystone of self-compassion.

Self-kindness is a slight proposal that we are deserving of our very own love together with treatment, especially in minutes of trouble or trouble. It starts off evolving by spotting humankind in addition to all its intricacies and additionally blemishes. As against rough self-complaint, self-kindness welcomes us to just accept ourselves with inflammation plus approval.

In the approach of self-kindness little motions of empathy can produce sizeable influences. It might consist of providing ourselves words of motivation as well as affirmation commemorating our successes, or merely expanding a minute of silent convenience to our worn-out hearts. With acts of self-kindness, we aid the seeds of compassion within, developing a far deeper feeling of link in addition to fitness.

Self-kindness also requires establishing limits together with focusing on our very own requirements and health. It suggests mentioning no to duties or dedications that drain our strength plus certainly to those who renew our spirit. By recognizing our limits, we understand ourselves confirming our fundamental worth as well as well worth.

In moments of warfare or trouble, self-kindness will become our supporting light. As opposed to bothering ourselves with our viewed failings, we provide ourselves the same poise and additional knowledge we'd in reality use for a cherished near buddy.

Through the lens of self-kindness, we see our difficulties not as symptoms of weak points, but as possibilities for development as well as expertise. Exercising self-kindness is not constantly easy, especially in a globe that usually highlights efficiency and also fulfillment maximum of all else. Nevertheless, it stays in minutes of self-doubt coupled with susceptibility that self-kindness beams brightest, providing us remedy as well as help among lifestyle's instabilities.

In welcoming self-kindness, we begin an experience of self-discovery in conjunction with recuperation. We find out to befriend ourselves with steadfast kindness and additionally compassion helping a deep feeling of love in addition to approval from inside. Via the slight welcome of self-kindness, we stir up the appeal and energy of our actual selves. Getting Rid of Self-Criticism and Negative Self-Talk: Within the targeted phase of Nurturing Self-Compassion, an important area offers the obstacle of Overcoming Self-Criticism and also Negative Self-Talk.

This part of the phase delves into techniques focused on disassembling harmful internal discussions and promoting an additional thoughtful self-view.

Unfavorable self-talk regularly comes from deep-rooted styles that could weaken fine self-image and prevent character improvement. In this zone, we find out the origins along with the influence of self-grievance acknowledging that minutes of trouble provide chances for prolonging compassion to ourselves in preference to succumbing to negativeness.

The walk inside the course of self-compassion includes acknowledging as well as trying out altered thoughts that maintain destructive self-talk. By inspecting the credibility of crucial ideas and additionally rewarding them with even more well-balanced viewpoints, visitors can proactively improve their inner stories and promote a kinder in addition to encouraging self-speak.

Mindfulness techniques play a vital obligation in this phase, functioning as a powerful device for dealing with unfavorable self-talk. By growing conscious know-how of thoughts and additionally feelings without judgment, humans can produce a place for self-compassion to grow. This approach motivates a non-reactive and also approving position inside the path of one's internal stories.

Furthermore, seeking out assistance is burdened as a vital part of disposing of self-grievance. Relied on buddies, members of the own family, or psychological health professionals can assist, and recognize, in addition to motivation during difficult instances. By connecting for assistance humans improve their sturdiness and benefit from useful understandings right into countering destructive self-communicate.

This segment does not intend to eliminate all traces of self-criticism but instead seems to sell considerate movement to at least one's internal battles. Accepting self-compassion finally ends up being a tool for browsing self-doubt in addition to an objection, advertising and marketing an additional favorable in addition to supporting partnership with oneself. As traffic is worried with these techniques, they begin a transformative ride within the path of getting rid of self-criticism, advertising, and marketing durability, plus supporting a far extra worrying self-view.

Mercy: Letting Go of Resentment and also Guilt. Within the greater comprehensive expedition of Nurturing Self-Compassion, an extensive emphasis pushes the transformative motif of Forgiveness: Letting Go of Resentment and additionally Guilt. In this element, we discover the impactful technique of mercy, stressing its function in selling self-compassion plus psychological recuperation.

Mercy is a person's journey along with the launch of animosity, rage, and remorse both within the course of oneself and others. Its capabilities as a course to internal tranquillity as well as psychological flexibility. At its significance, mercy is an act of self-compassion, along with the growth of generosity as well as expertise oneself for preceding mistakes at the side of considered drawbacks.

The technique of mercy encompasses oneself to comprise others, acknowledging mankind and additionally fallibility fundamental in everybody. It does no longer excuse vicious activities however instead equips human beings to get better their freedom, rejecting to be targeted using preceding injuries or lawsuits.

A vital facet of mercy is discharging remorse usually rooted in outlandish standards or harping on previous remorse. Via self-compassion in addition to a recognition of essential worthiness, people can launch the hassle of remorse, paving the manner for internal tranquillity collectively with self-forgiveness. While mercy is probably difficult in addition to needing time as well as mental dealing, its rewards-- liberty from psychological problems, inner tranquillity restored self-compassion are sizeable. By welcoming mercy people begin a ride of self-discovery and recuperation together with permission developing further compassion and launching partnerships with themselves as well as others. As visitors are concerned with the transformative method of mercy, they open themselves to countless opportunities for self-compassion recuperation, and additionally revival.

Chapter Four

Prioritizing Self-Care

In the quest for self-love in addition to alternative well-being, the segment Prioritizing Self-Care unravels as a critical expedition of the transformative duty self-care performs in our lives. Identifying the cost of self-care as an important want, we explore the diverse measurements of this approach and address functional understandings for incorporating it right into our everyday regimens.

Self-care usually misconstrued as a high-quit, arises as a vital device for keeping equilibrium and additionally energy amongst lifestyle's desires. This segment intends to redefine self-care past plain extravagance, stressing its obligation to aid physical, mental, and mental well-being.

The concept of self-care is provided as a tailor-made in addition to a calculated approach. Viewers are stimulated to begin a ride of self-discovery spotting their distinct requirements in addition to picks. This system units the shape for generating a tailored self-care normal that straightens with a personal way of existence plus concerns.

Variety in self-care strategies takes the highlight recognizing that health is numerous. Exercise, mindfulness techniques progressive searches in addition to supporting social hyperlinks are looked at as important factors of an in-depth self-care toolkit. Functional suggestions and additional hints are given, encouraging visitors to weave a selection of self-care strategies properly into their lives.

Within the context of self-care, the facility of wholesome and balanced borders emerges as a recurring fashion. Establishing and additionally keeping limits ends up being an effective manner of defensive man or woman time, strength in addition to psychological regions. The section highlights the cost of saying no when required, allowing humans to be aware of self-care without regret or doubt.

Resolving regular demanding situations to self-care consisting of time restrictions plus out-of-door assumptions this phase equips viewers with procedures for putting off demanding situations. The recognition exists on promoting one's well-being collectively by making calculated alternatives that straighten with the search for self-love.

Via interaction with the understandings collectively with techniques detailed in this section, traffic is welcome to begin a transformative ride. Prioritizing self-care ends up being a cornerstone for cultivating a far extra properly balanced, satisfying, in addition to worrying partnership with oneself. In welcoming self-care, humans develop sturdiness plus empowerment, browsing life's barriers with a restored complacency of properly being in addition to self-love.

The Duty of Self-Care in Self-Love: Self-care is the keystone of supporting self-love a crucial area in the more complete day trip of alternative well-being. In comprehending the good-sized partnership between self-care and also self-love we begin an experience of planned as well as transformative methods.

Specifying Self-Care as Fundamental: Self-care is reframed as a non-negotiable technique crucial for assisting bodily, mental, and also psychological well-being. It is going beyond the arena of extravagance, finishing up being useful willpower to apprehend and additionally cognizance of one's wellness.

Alternative Well-Being: Accepting an alternative standpoint, self-care is attended to be a nicely-rounded approach to resolving numerous measurements of health. It consists of physical activities mindfulness techniques, creative ventures, and additionally assisting social links, promoting a detailed feeling of vigor as well as equilibrium.

Customization of Self-Care: Readers are welcomed right into a trip of self-discovery, acknowledging their wonderful demands, alternatives, and additional limits. The phase stresses the significance of crafting an individualized self-care routine customized to a particular way of residing plus concerns making certain sustainability and additional verbal exchange.

Boundaries and also Saying No: A principal motif arises around the facility of healthful and balanced limits. By welcoming the strength of no people gain returned employer over their time plus electricity selling a society of self-worth mixed with permission inside their self-care strategies.

Getting Rid of Barriers: Attending to regular challenges such as time restrictions and also public assumptions visitors are outfitted with functional tactics for disposing of limitations to self-care. Encouraging people to promote their nicely-being the section instills a feeling of the enterprise as well as durability in navigating limitations.

Transformative Impact: Self-care is proclaimed as a transformative driving force on the path of self-love. Via planned acts of self-nurturing in addition to compassion, human beings develop a far deeper feeling of approval, and durability together with inner tranquillity. Self-care comes to be a spiritual recurring, helping the seeds of self-love inside.

Accepting Self-Care as a Ritual: In a shutting invite, traffic is encouraged to welcome self-care as a religious ordinary of self-love. By recognizing the widespread hyperlink between calculated self-care strategies and the boom of self-love humans begin a journey of vast improvement along with permission.

In this specific expedition, the sector brightens the vital interaction between self-care and self-love. With calculated methods and additionally transformative understandings human beings locate the transformative ability of self-care as a path to welcoming in addition to commemorating the significance of self-love in all its measurements.

Producing a Personalized Self-Care Routine: Starting the journey to broaden a tailored self-care routine includes a considerate expedition of your specific requirements and alternatives alongside health. This technique unravels permitting you to customise self-care techniques to straighten effects with the details of your existence.

Start with a deep examination of self-discovery, participating in reflective workout routines to show what reverberates with your genuine self. Check out obligations that deliver you a sense of delight, entertainment, and gratification.

Recognize your middle necessities through bodily, psychological, along mental measurements. This motion wishes a sincere evaluation of locations in your lifestyles that want help coupled with attention. Prioritize those necessities as you lay the structure for your self-care routine.

Think approximately the context of your manner of dwelling, regimens, and also concerns while customizing your self-care methods. The goal is to include self-care effects properly into your life, making certain that it continues to be both possible and lasting.

Accept a nicely balanced technique by way of inclusive of a selection of tasks that satisfy diverse factors of fitness. Incorporate sports that assist your body, mindfulness techniques for mental exceptional, imaginative searches for psychological expression in addition to social links for relational pride.

Develop workouts within your self-care regimen to consist of a feeling of connection plus intentionality. Rituals may be as easy as an early morning mindfulness method as soon as per week self-care day, or any kind of every day that brings a feeling of based totally in addition to an objective.

Infuse happiness properly into your self-care routine with the aid of that specialize in duties that convey pleasure coupled with delight. Take element in leisure activities and enjoy minutes of pure delight coupled with included aspects that cause exhilaration.

Preserve versatility and additionally versatility in your self-care technique acknowledging the colourful nature of lifestyles. Be open to readjusting your regular based totally upon changing situations, necessities, and additional concerns. Routinely sign up in your personal to examine the performance of your self-care routine.

Assess what's functioning well plus take into consideration adjustments or refinements to a long way better preserve your health. Commemorate your willpower to self-nurturing methods and also apprehend the progression you make on this ride toward self-love and opportunity fitness.

Chapter Five

Structure Self-confidence as well as Self-belief

The phase of structuring a nice self-photograph plus self-confidence probes deep into the complex process of assisting a favorable self-photograph plus inner guarantee. It is an experience of self-discovery, self-reputation, and improvement that equips people to welcome their essential well-being and additional capacities.

At the coronary heart of this section exists the acknowledgment that self-worth and also self-assurance are essential columns of wellness plus achievement. With a detailed expedition of different approaches in addition to principles viewers start a transformative ride towards growing a healthy and balanced long-lasting feeling of self.

The experience starts with self-consciousness welcoming site visitors to find out their thoughts, ideas in addition to feelings regarding themselves.
By cultivating an understanding plus a non-judgmental understanding in their inner globe people outline for self-discovery coupled with approval.

Main to the system is the approach of self-compassion, which features as a mild helping light in minutes of self-question plus objection. With self-compassion, human beings find out to welcome their imperfections at the side of treating themselves with kindness as well as understanding, selling a much deeper feeling of self-regard plus approval.

The segment highlights the value of checking out self-proscribing thoughts in addition to changing them with encouragement in addition to putting forward thoughts. By reframing negative self-communicate and developing a good frame of thought, we, human beings harness the strength of self-communicate as a device for supporting self-confidence and also self-confidence.

A crucial element of structure self-assurance and additionally self-confidence is the farming of durability when faced with challenges as well as problems. Viewers are encouraged to simply accept failings as possibilities for improvement in addition to coming across, and acknowledging that power is developed with determination in addition to a tremendous outlook.

The section discovers useful techniques for reinforcing self-esteem together with self-confidence in distinctive domains of existence, which include partnerships, jobs, and additionally personal targets. From organizing obtainable purposes to commemorating successes, humans discover to develop a sense of talent in addition to the competencies of their ventures.

Throughout the phase, the price of self-care arises as a persisting motif. Focusing on one's bodily, mental, and also psychological fitness is important for developing a good self-image and internal self-belief. By exercising self-care routines as well as useful oneself, people replace their inner resources as well as develop a feeling of energy collectively with sturdiness.

As the experience unravels, visitors are welcomed to welcome susceptibility as a direction to credibility as well as a hyperlink. By welcoming their true selves in addition to owning their special toughness and additionally high features human beings grow a deep feeling of self-assurance as well as self-belief of their worthiness.

To sum this up, it shapes wonderful self-photo in addition to self-assurance acts as a plan for individual development at the side of empowerment. It is a journey of self-discovery, self-attractiveness, and self-empowerment that equips people to welcome their actual selves as well as stay actually with self-confidence and poise.

Commending Your Achievements and Additional Successes: Nestled in the wider expedition of structure self-worth plus self-assurance a vital segment lights up the technique of Celebrating Your Achievements in addition to Successes. This area acknowledges the transformative electricity of acknowledging coupled with spotting a person's success as a vital action towards growing a positive self-photograph.

The journey starts evolved with an alternate in the body of mind advising site visitors to develop a practice of recognizing their achievement regardless of exactly how little. By making the effort to evaluate fulfillment, people confirm their skills together with including the muse of a high-quality self-photo.

The zone looks into the art of establishing available functions plus turning factors. By simplifying bigger goals right into conceivable moves, human beings produce opportunities for fulfillment that may be diagnosed as well as honored alongside the street. This approach now not simplest complements self-belief but also elements a substantial measure of progression.

In addition, the approach of commemorating successes is going beyond outdoor recognition. Visitors are stimulated to internalize and feel their tasks figuring out the determination, strength, in addition to capability related to their accomplishments. This indoor recognition comes to be a powerful aid of self-belief in addition to self-assurance.

The phase highlights the significance of growing a positive partnership with achievement. By reframing success as a ride rather than a vicinity human beings find to cost the non-stop process of development in addition to discovery. Each success regardless of exactly how tiny finally ends up being an affidavit to individual growth collectively with sturdiness.

As the arena unravels site visitors are offered distinct techniques for commemorating their successes. Whether through self-reflection, journaling, or sharing success with trusted proper pals the act of occasion comes to be a routine that complements favorable self-talk as well as self-appreciation.

Essentially, Celebrating Your Achievements in conjunction with Success involves a transformative technique in the greater comprehensive shape of structure self-worth as well as self-assurance. It encourages people to transport their emphasis from regarded drawbacks to massive success growing a resistant plus favorable self-perception that comes to be a keystone of their experience closer to self-confidence and also self-confidence.

Obstructing Limiting Beliefs: Within the intricate tapestry of shape self-belief plus self-confidence, an intensive excursion unfurls in the sort of Challenging Limiting Beliefs: This area appears into the complex panorama of our thoughts welcoming viewers to research at the side of enhance the thoughts that would preclude their complacency at the side of self-belief.

The journey starts evolved with self-cognizance motivating human beings to listen to their internal dialogue. Viewers are influenced to understand as well as apprehend thoughts that sabotage their self-confidence or hold a destructive self-photo. By radiating a mild on those limiting ideas, human beings lay the foundation for improvement.

Central to the system is the technique of self-compassion. As traffic assignments restrict ideas, they're directed to come back near themselves with generosity and additional expertise. The goal isn't always to slam however to cultivate an encouraging as well as considerate inner dialogue that leads the way for self-discovery as well as development.

The segment highlights the energy of reframing unfavorable self-talk. Viewers are motivated to protect the credibility of restricting ideas collectively by changing them by way of motivating and additionally verifying ideas. This includes doubting the evidence maintaining these ideas coupled with looking for exchange viewpoints that straighten with their real capabilities and also capacity.

Cognitive restructuring finally ends up being a crucial facet of checking out limiting thoughts. By spotting cognitive distortions inclusive of catastrophizing or overgeneralization, humans find out how to enhance their assumed styles. This involves purposely moving from a destructive collectively with a self-defeating manner of wandering to an extra nicely balanced as well as affordable point of view.

The excursion encompasses the beginnings of restricting ideas welcoming viewers to review the resource of those thoughts. Whether embedded in preceding experiences social assumptions, or contrasts with others recognizing the start of proscribing ideas resources understandings right into their nature and additionally uses a route to take them apart.

Sensible strategies for checking out proscribing thoughts are woven right into the tale. From favorable affirmations collectively with visualization techniques to seek out help from coaches or experts, people are endorsed to proactively participate in the process of enhancing their idea gadgets.

Throughout this segment, the fee of persistence plus uniformity is highlighted. Testing and proscribing thoughts is a continuous process that desires recurring initiative and also self-thinking.

We are encouraged to commemorate little achievements and understand progression, spotting that the journey towards building a wonderful self-picture together with self-confidence is marked through non-stop improvement.

Within the tapestry of positive self-photo and self-belief structure the functional sector of Setting Realistic Goals plus Taking Action; involves a hands-on evaluation, equipping human beings to browse the floor of goals coupled with high-quality progression.

1. Clear up Your Aspirations:
Start by making clean your passions. Assess your worth, and interests, collectively with places of individual development. Specify certain objectives that reverberate along with your actual self-straightening with both your goals and gift conditions.

2. Make Your Goals SMART:
Change your desires right into SMART dreams- Specific, Measurable, Achievable Relevant as well as Time-Bound. This crucial shape ensures quality making your targets enormous in addition to providing a development plan. As an example, in preference to an unclear goal light workout lots greater to opt for a SMART goal like strolling for 30 minutes every early morning.

3. Break Down Larger Goals:
Big targets may be hard. Damage them down properly into smaller-sized or achievable jobs. By unwinding the journey right into practical movements, you produce a sense of fulfillment with each activity completed, selling a good feedback loophole for your self-esteem.

4. Grow a Growth Mindset:
Accept difficulties with an evolved way of wondering. Sight obstacles aren't as failings but as probabilities to find out as well as great-track your approach. This way of thinking modifications settings limitations as critical parts of the ride, including on your man or woman and additionally psychological development.

5. Take on Deliberate coupled with regular Action:
Relocate from instruction to pastime. Take calculated as well as constant moves in the direction of your goals. Whether it is committing a certain time every day to a career activity or

integrating new practices gradually, wilful activities produce a sense of firmness in addition to fulfillment.

6. Accept Micro-Actions:
Incorporate the precept of micro-actions properly into your regimen. These are tiny attainable jobs that upload to your larger objective. The advancing effect of regular micro-movements constructs strength, enhancing your willpower in addition to improving yourself-belief.

7. Discover in addition to Adapt:
Approach your journey with a knowing mindset. Consistently examine your development to determine what jobs are properly, and additionally agree to modify your technique if required. Picking up from stories, each success plus barriers makes sure a vibrant collectively advancing course closer to your goals.

8. Commemorate Progress:
Commemorate now not simply the accomplishment of the closing targets but likewise the development made along the street. Recognize your projects in addition to achievements, irrespective of precisely how little. This favorable helps bureaucracy a story of achievement, including a dramatic boom of yourself-belief.

Establishing Realistic Goals plus Taking Action is a plan that urges deliberate, calculated actions within the course of a person's passions. By integrating these useful standards properly into your ride, you no longer need to move on however moreover grow a long-lasting and additionally superb feeling of self-alongside the road.

Chapter Six

Cultivating Appreciation Together with Mindfulness: Nurturing Inner Health.

The degree of increasing recognition plus mindfulness untwines as an adventure proper into the transformative globes of gift-minute reputation in addition to a reputation for the riches in our lives. This ride overviews humans inside the path of inner tranquillity and longevity plus an intensive hyperlink with both themselves as well as the globe around them.

Comprehending Gratitude: The segment begins by way of penetrating the relevance of appreciation-- a recognition of the blessings and additional wealth fundamental in our lives. Visitors are prompted to discover how thankfulness can boost their ordinary stories rousing a favorable and appreciative point of view.

Working Out Mindfulness: At its core mindfulness takes the spotlight advising human beings to develop a useful know-how of the here-and-now minute. Via mindfulness techniques inclusive of mirrored images, and deep respiration paired with sensory reputation visitors find out to floor themselves inside the contemporary without judgment or disturbances.

Sustaining Inner Well-being: Central to the growth of gratitude in addition to mindfulness is the nursing of internal health. Organizing self-care comes to be a keystone in welcoming site visitors to apprehend their mental and psychological necessities with compassion coupled with compassion. This self-nurturing lays the foundation for ample admiration and additionally mindfulness in regular lifestyles.

Approving Acceptance: Mindfulness offers the precept of approval-- an invitation to meet every minute with life at the side of non-resistance. With approval, humans find out to welcome each other the pride plus difficulties of existence marketing a feeling of neutrality plus tranquillity within the middle of the ups and also downs of stories.

Improving Connection: Thanks, works as an extensive bridge, increasing links with oneself, others as well as the globe. By cultivating an attitude of admiration website traffic boosts their partnerships, develops situations, and additionally in reality senses a heightened feeling of relatedness with the precise Internet of life.

Expanding Resilience: Mindfulness plus thankfulness entwine as effective devices for developing energy. Securing oneself in the here and now minute plus valuing the real advantages within the middle of the problem flowers a durable spirit encouraging humans to browse lifestyles' difficulties with elegance and additional nerve.

Fostering a Positive Mindset: In harmony popularity plus mindfulness put it up for sale a favorable evaluation— a lens through which human beings watch the globe with visibility, inquisitiveness coupled with admiration. This favorable expectation changes boundaries right into opportunities for development instilling life with definition together with function.

Including Practices into Daily Life: The segment wraps up with the aid of providing sensible strategies for without difficulty incorporating thankfulness as well as mindfulness strategies properly into life.

Staying in these days' Minutes: The level of residing within the here and now min unwinds as a journey right into mindfulness in addition to the complete art of approving the present. It invites people to release the fears of the beyond plus the demanding situations of destiny, main them in the direction of a state of vast presence at the side of entertainment.

Staying within the here-and-now minute begins with the development of conscious information. Visitors are entreated to deliver their hobby to today's revel in, enjoying the perspectives, seems, and emotions bordering them. With mindfulness, people find out to steady themselves in wealth these days.

Stress and tension regarding destiny generally draw hobbies far from the present. The phase overviews people in browsing unpredictability with the aid of concentrating on what they could adjust inside the right here and now. Via mindfulness, viewers discover beforehand near destiny with a primarily based and additionally calm point of view.

Thankfulness involves a transformative approach to the art of dwelling within the existing. Visitors are welcome to price the little, ordinary minutes similarly to locating pleasure in primary delight. By developing thankfulness people enhance their social links with the present marketing a feeling of delight mixed with wealth.

Residing in the latest minute has to do with instilling mindfulness proper into everyday responsibilities. Whether it is delighting in a dish, walking, or taking components in resourceful searches, visitors are stimulated to exist and submerged within the enjoyment. This conscious interplay amplifies the wealth of each minute.

The present-second dwelling consists of social links. The segment discovers the relevance of being present in discussions, growing tons of deeper links with others. With lively attention coupled with real participation, human beings domesticate purposeful partnerships that have grown in wealth in recent times.

Staying in the here and now incorporates expanding compassion for oneself. The phase discovers the method of conscious self-compassion motivating people to treat themselves with kindness along understanding. By welcoming one's susceptibilities plus defects, people develop a nurturing internal atmosphere today.

The phase wraps up by motivating people to weave mindfulness right into the material of their way of life. From including conscious minutes right into everyday regimens to producing specialized areas for representation visitors are motivated to promote a continual method of residing in today.

Basically "Living in the Present Moment" ends up being an overview of tranquility plus contentment. By inviting conscious understanding along with growing thankfulness people launch a transformative trip towards a much more conscious plus improving presence in the here and now.

Chapter Seven

Fostering Healthy Relationships: Nurturing Connection Along with Well-being

The exploration of nurturing wholesome relationships untangles as an experience proper into the traits of the hyperlink, interplay in addition to shared nicely-being. This section overviews people towards growing functional links with others, stressing the relevance of compassion. Efficient interplay coupled with not-unusual improvement.

Structure Empathy is highlighted as an essential detail motivating humans to establish a deep expertise of others' viewpoints, and sensations, collectively with stories. By growing compassion, human beings produce a shape for actual links alongside shared assistance. Reliable Communication is highlighted as a keystone of healthy and balanced connections. The section focuses on the art of efficient interaction, highlighting lively interest, clean expression of ideas, and also sensations together with the capability to browse disputes favorably. These abilities add to developing know-how and also developing more powerful links.

Developing Boundaries is observed as a crucial component of keeping wholesome and balanced partnerships. Viewers are motivated to set up in addition to regard limits, making positive that people experience blanketed and also valued within the connection. This phase overviews people in locating stability that advertises self-reliance as well as connections.

Nurturing Trust is decided as the keystone of healthful and balanced partnerships. The excursion untangles the traits of structure coupled with retaining the accept as true with a fund with openness, and integrity alongside open interaction. Depend on flourishes a sense of protection and protection as well as affection, developing a regular shape for the development of the connection.

Shared targets are recognized as important for healthy and balanced partnerships. Visitors are stimulated to find out compatibility in center ideas, and goals together with their way of lifestyles. This day trip assists humans develop links with those that associate with their important concepts, selling a mile deeper feeling of connection plus function.

Growth within connections is highlighted as an essential facet. Healthy and balanced hyperlinks enable humans inside the region in conjunction with assistance to go after individual development as well as desires adding to the general well-being of each person within the connection.

Navigating Challenges Together is pressured as a collective initiative. The segment overviews humans in encountering barriers as a group highlighting synergy resilience, as well as efficient hassle-fixing. Healthy and balanced connections are better with shared projects to put off barriers.

Commemorating Achievements is identified as vital to developing a favorable coupled with encouraging environment. The segment urges traffic to proactively discover and commemorate each other's turning factors adding to a society of recognition and motivation.

Balancing Independence and Togetherness is identified as crucial for a healthy relationship. The bankruptcy explores the significance of keeping personal identities whilst playing shared reviews. This stability guarantees that each partners feel fulfilled and valued in the relationship.

In essence, Fostering Healthy Relationships serves as a guide to constructing connections that uplift, nurture, and make contributions to the well-being of all individuals concerned. Through empathy, effective verbal exchange, consideration, shared values, and a commitment to growth, individuals embark on a journey toward relationships that are pleasurable, harmonious, and enduring.

Setting Healthy Boundaries in Relationships: In the world of healthy relationships, placing limitations is important. This includes organizing clear limits that appreciate a person's needs and promote a feeling of protection and admiration in the dating. It's a delicate stability that guarantees each independence and connection, fostering a dynamic wherein individuals feel valued and understood.

Assertive and Respectful Communication: In the artwork of healthful verbal exchange, getting to know assertiveness and recognition is pivotal. Assertive verbal exchange entails expressing thoughts and emotions in reality and confidently, fostering open dialogue. Simultaneously, respecting others' views guarantees a collaborative and expert environment inside relationships, laying the groundwork for powerful and harmonious interactions.

Surrounding Yourself with Supportive Individuals: Cultivating a Positive Circle In the pursuit of well-being, consciously selecting a supportive circle will become paramount. This includes surrounding yourself with folks that uplift, encourage, and recognize your adventure. A supportive community offers emotional sustenance, practical advice, and a feeling of belonging. It involves cultivating relationships that contribute positively to your boom and fostering an environment wherein mutual guidance prospers. Choosing a supportive circle is an intentional step closer to constructing a community that enhances your typical well-being and resilience.

Chapter Eight

Overcoming Obstacles on the Path to Self-Love

Here we embark on a deep and nuanced adventure, delving into the intricacies of overcoming limitations on the profound path to self-love. This pivotal chapter serves as a complete guide, providing a wealth of insights and realistic techniques to navigate the demanding situations that regularly accompany the pursuit of an extra profound connection with oneself.

At its core, the chapter initiates through unraveling the layers of inner resistance that people may also encounter. It delves into the roots of self-doubt, fear, and ingrained beliefs, presenting readers with a reflective space to recognize the inner dynamics that could act as obstacles to self-love. This preliminary exploration lays the foundation for a greater profound understanding of the self.

External impacts, and some other sizable aspects, are intricately examined within this chapter. Societal expectancies, cultural norms, and the impact of relationships on self-notion are explored in detail. Readers's advantage of precious insights into navigating external pressures whilst preserving authenticity, empowering them to shape a shallowness adventure aligned with their genuine selves.

A poignant subject matter woven into this chapter is the embrace of vulnerability. The resistance regularly felt toward vulnerability is explored with intensity and sensitivity. Readers are guided through the transformative power of beginning up to one's authentic self, highlighting vulnerability as a gateway to profound self-popularity and love.

Past traumas, emotional wounds that could solidly shadow in the course of self-love, are unraveled in this exploration. The segment offers practical strategies for recovery and self-compassion, empowering readers to navigate and release the load of past stories, and fostering an extra compassionate relationship with oneself.

Patience and self-kindness turn out to be essential virtues all through the chapter. The significance of cultivating those characteristics is explored, providing realistic exercises and attitude shifts to foster a compassionate internal speak. Readers are equipped to navigate setbacks with resilience and gentleness, spotting that self-love is a journey marked with the aid of progress instead of perfection.

A growth mindset, considered as a powerful tool for overcoming limitations, is unfolded with realistic strategies for cultivation. The bankruptcy courses readers into embracing demanding situations as possibilities for private growth, instilling a mindset that aligns setbacks with the transformative journey toward self-love.

The position of self-care practices is underscored, encompassing mindfulness strategies and nurturing physical well-being. These practices are offered as anchors, providing people with the resilience needed to face and overcome demanding situations. The chapter invites readers to discover a whole lot of self-care techniques that resonate with their precise wishes and options.

Acknowledging the importance of searching for expert aid, the chapter delves into the advantages of remedy, counseling, or coaching. Readers are guided on the way to navigate these sources, leveraging professional guidance to conquer unique limitations and deepen their journey to self-love.

This chapter concludes by clarifying the issue of patience in self-love situations. Readers are empowered to see obstacles not as obstacles but as obstacles, contributing to their sense of evolution. Building resilience becomes a transformative part of the ongoing journey of self-love, reinforcing the idea that challenges are important parts of growth and self-discovery.

This chapter stands as a rich and complex guide, providing readers with a comprehensive toolkit to navigate and overcome the many obstacles we encounter on the complex and transformative path of loving yourself.

Chapter Nine

Embracing Self-Love as a Lifelong Journey

In the dynamics of private growth and well-being, one needs to include self-love as a long-lasting adventure. This expertise serves as a guiding mild, illuminating the route toward a deeper and greater enduring connection with oneself.

At its middle, embrace self-love no longer as a vacation spot but as an ongoing, lifelong journey. It challenges conventional notions of success and fulfillment, emphasizing that self-love isn't an intention to be attained but a state of being to be nurtured and cultivated through the years.

Throughout life, we're encouraged to embody the inherent imperfections and complexities of the shallowness adventure. We well know that self-love isn't linear and that setbacks and challenges are inevitable along the way. Instead of viewing those limitations as screw-ups, readers are endorsed to see them as opportunities for boom and self-discovery.

A principal subject matter woven in the course of this bankruptcy is the importance of self-compassion. Readers are reminded to treat themselves with kindness and understanding, especially during instances of war or adversity. Self-compassion will become a guiding precept, imparting solace and aid as people navigate the highs and lows in their self-love journey.

We also explore the idea of self-recognition as a cornerstone of self-love. Readers are recommended to cultivate a deep knowledge of their very own desires, desires, and values. Through introspection and mirrored image, individuals benefit from readability approximately who they are and what brings them pleasure and success, laying the foundation for a greater authentic and significant life. Another key factor of this subject is the belief of forgiveness and letting cross of the past. Readers are invited to release the burdens of resentment, guilt, and self-blame which can weigh them down. By practicing forgiveness, individuals unfastened themselves from the shackles of the past, allowing space for recovery and growth to flourish.

We also emphasize the importance of self-care as a foundational practice in the journey toward self-love. Readers are recommended to prioritize their bodily, emotional, and mental well-being, recognizing that self-care is not egocentric but important for personal flourishing.

As we draw to a close, we are reminded that self-love is a dynamic and ever-evolving method. It calls for patience, determination, and a willingness to embody vulnerability. But especially, it needs authenticity—the courage to be proper to oneself and to honor one's real worth and dignity.

In essence, this serves as a beacon of desire and suggestion, reminding readers that self-love isn't always a destination but a sacred adventure—one that unfolds with grace and intentionality, leading in the direction of an extra profound experience of wholeness, success, and pleasure.

Embracing Change and Growth: A Narrative Unveiling: Within the tapestry of private improvement, this narrative unfolds, weaving a wealthy exploration across the transformative topics of exchange and growth. It invites readers right into a dynamic interplay between lifestyles' evolution and the potential for profound non-public and spiritual maturation.

At its core, the narrative activates readers to shift their perspective on change, urging them to embrace it as an indispensable and herbal side of existence's unfolding journey. The concept is gently woven that within life's transitions lie possibilities for learning, edition, and the cultivation of a greater enriched, significant existence.

The journey of personal and spiritual growth takes center level, navigating the multifaceted dimensions of emotional expansiveness, intellectual curiosity, and non-secular evolution. Readers are beckoned to embark on a private odyssey, unlocking the inherent capability for chronic improvement.

A resonant subject woven in the course of this is the brave act of stepping past consolation zones. Embracing alternate and fostering growth frequently calls for venturing into the unknown. Profound increase and transformation, the narrative shows, regularly emerge from the soreness and uncertainty inherent in the process of change.

The narrative takes a contemplative pause to explore strategies for cultivating resilience, encouraging readers to understand obstacles as gateways to increase. Resilience emerges as a steadfast best friend, empowering individuals to navigate the undulating currents of life with grace and internal strength.

Self-reflection turns into a poignant thread, inviting people to embark on an adventure of introspection. Through reflective practices, individuals gain a deeper understanding of their values, aspirations, and areas for improvement. This self-focus is portrayed as a guiding compass, steering people towards effective and transformative trade.

Mindfulness infuses the narrative with an invitation to appreciate the existing second. Cultivating a heightened awareness permits people to relish the nuances of the evolving adventure. Within the canvas of aware dwelling, people discover solace and wisdom, allowing them to gracefully navigate the transitions of existence.

As we sum up, there may be a palpable sense of empowerment—a recognition that trade is not a pressure to be resisted but a dynamic catalyst for high-quality transformation. By immersing themselves in the difficult dance of embracing exchange and seeking growth, individuals embark on a soul-stirring adventure closer to a lifestyle that is not most effective but resilient but authentically enjoyable.

Inspiring Others to Love Themselves: A Detailed Exploration: In the sweet journey of personal development, there exists a profound opportunity to encourage and uplift others on their journey to self-love. This certain exploration illuminates the pathways and concepts through which individuals can emerge as beacons of encouragement and empowerment, igniting the flames of self-love in the ones around them.

At its middle, inspiring others to love themselves starts with embodying authenticity and vulnerability. Individuals who authentically proportion their self-love journey create a safe and relatable area for others to discover and include their paths to self-discovery and popularity.

Empathy emerges as a cornerstone in this undertaking, as people seek to apprehend and connect to the stories and emotions of others. By listening deeply and offering compassionate guidance, individuals can domesticate a sense of belonging and validation, fostering an environment wherein self-love can flourish.

An essential factor of inspiring self-love in others entails celebrating their inherent worth and distinctiveness. By recognizing and affirming the strengths, skills, and characteristics of those around them, individuals assist in cultivating a sense of self-value and appreciation, laying the groundwork for a deeper feeling of self-love.

Practicing lively encouragement and validation becomes a transformative tool in this journey. By offering sincere praise and recognition for the achievements and progress of others, individuals empower them to recognize their worth and capability, fostering a fine self-image and shallowness.

The exploration delves into the strength of modeling self-compassion and self-care as acts of love closer to oneself. By prioritizing their well-being and demonstrating healthful boundaries and self-care practices, people inspire others to prioritize their self-love and nourishment.

Authenticity and transparency emerge as guiding principles in inspiring others to like themselves. By sharing their personal struggles, challenges, and triumphs with honesty and vulnerability, people create areas for others to feel visible, heard, and understood, fostering a deep sense of connection and attractiveness.

The narrative also underscores the significance of fostering a growth-oriented mindset in others. By encouraging resilience, self-reflection, and a willingness to embrace change and growth, individuals empower others to navigate their self-love journey with braveness, resilience, and charm.

As the discourse comes to a close, there is a profound popularity of the transformative impact that people will have in inspiring others to like themselves. By embodying authenticity, empathy, celebration, encouragement, and self-compassion, people grow to be catalysts for tremendous trade, igniting the flames of self-love and empowerment inside the hearts of those around them.

Conclusion

In the journey of self-love, we have traversed a profound panorama of introspection, boom, and transformation. As we finish this book, it's vital to reflect on the myriad insights, revelations, and reviews that have illuminated our course toward extra self-reputation and compassion.

Throughout these pages, we have delved deep into the complex layers of self-discovery, exploring the complexities of our innermost thoughts, emotions, and ideals. We've confronted the shadows of self-doubt and insecurity, and in doing so, we've unearthed the seeds of resilience and electricity that lie within us.

We have learned that self-love is not a vacation spot to be reached but a non-stop journey—a journey marked via moments of triumph and moments of battle, moments of readability and moments of misunderstanding. It's an adventure that requires courage, vulnerability, and unwavering commitment to our well-being and happiness.

As we have navigated this journey, we have encountered useful companions along the way—partners who've walked beside us, providing their knowledge, empathy, and unwavering support. We've located the profound energy of connection, knowing that in sharing our stories, our struggles, and our triumphs, we create a tapestry of empathy and expertise that binds us collectively in cohesion and compassion.

We have come to apprehend that self-love isn't always a solitary pursuit but a collective enterprise—a shared dedication to honoring and celebrating the inherent worth and dignity of each individual. It's a dedication to building communities of reputation and inclusion, wherein all people are seen, valued, and embraced for who they may be. As we bid farewell to these pages, let us deliver forward the lessons we've discovered and the insights we have won into our daily lives. Let us cultivate a practice of self-love that extends past the limits of those words—an exercise rooted in kindness, forgiveness, and unconditional reputation.

May we consider that self-love isn't always about perfection however about embracing our imperfections with grace and compassion. May we honor the adventure—the highs and the lows, the victories and the setbacks—as sacred milestones in the direction of our fulfillment and self-awareness.

May we in no way forget that the finest act of love we can offer ourselves is the unwavering commitment to expose up, day by day, with an open coronary heart and a courageous spirit—to include ourselves fully and unapologetically, just as we are.

As we end, may all of us embark on this adventure with a renewed feeling of purpose and possibility. For in the adventure of self-love, the opportunities are infinite, and the rewards are endless.

Notes:

Notes:

References:

Discover the Art of

Self-Love

...Unleashing Your Brilliance, Embracing Your Worth!...

©

Copyright 2024

Peter K. Ndung'u

All rights reserved.

For more information contact:

Phone; +254 72283 5564/+254-7246 57794

Email:kiruuz@gmail.com

www.ingramcontent.com/pod-product-compliance
Lightning Source LLC
Chambersburg PA
CBHW070821280726
48660CB00017B/2379